Peripheral Neuropathy 101: A Guide For Patients

By Dr. Naota Hashimoto

First Edition

ISBN 978-1508696131

Printed in the United States of America

Table of Contents

Introduction

This book, *A Doctor's Guide To Peripheral Neuropathy* is two books in one, or rather it is one book printed twice.

The first (approx.) half is the book printed with normal lay-out conventions which makes it the easiest way for many people to read the book.

Peripheral Neuropathy, as you will learn, afflicts a wide range of people. A good many have their best eyesight behind them. To address this we have changed the lay-out and have adopted larger print and formatting rules that are the latest in easy to read type.

The book has then been reprinted, exactly, again.

The easy to read version begins on page 61.

Chapter 1: What is Neuropathy?

Neuropathy is a condition in which a person experiences pain and numbness often in the hands and feet, though it may occur in other parts of the body as well.

The word itself betrays the general and somewhat mysterious nature of the disease. Neuro- of or related to nerves and -pathy a disease or ailment of. In medical circles, one can see that a lot of different conditions could be attributed to "something wrong with the nerves".

Regardless of the vague definition, Peripheral Neuropathy sometimes referred to as Polyneuropathy, is typically diagnosed when a person has pain or numbness where there is no direct or observable cause for it.

The complication occurs as a result of nerve damage in the peripheral nervous system. There are 3 main types of nerves that can be involved:

Autonomic nerves: These regulate heart rate, sweating, blood pressure and other automatic functions of the body.

Motor nerves: Control the body muscles and are usually under conscious control.

Sensory nerves: These transmit sensations (such as information about heat and cold) from other body parts to the brain.

<u>Symptoms of Neuropathy</u>

Most people with Neuropathy often report feeling a tingling pain or burning sensation. Generally, an individual's specific symptoms may depend on the kind of nerves affected. Common symptoms and signs of Neuropathy include:

- Numbness and tingling sensation in, usually, the hands or feet but which can spread to the arms and legs. This sensation can make sleep very difficult.

- Sharp, electric-like pain.

- The sense that one is stepping off into nothing with each step.

- Burning pain where no burn has occurred. Often it is impossible to point to an exact source of the pain as it will seem to be in an entire area such as the whole foot.

- Muscle weakness /paralysis.

- Heat intolerance. Running one's hands under warm water may cause discomfort

- High sensitivity to touch. Even light brushes may prove to be very uncomfortable.

- Dizziness due to changes in the blood pressure. This often shows up when standing up after sitting for some time.

Causes of Neuropathy

Since the complication may be caused by different factors or a combination of factors, it is not easy to pinpoint its exact cause(s).

This fact is well known to many Neuropathy sufferers as they have often tried many different treatments.

There are certain factors, however, that are associated with development of Neuropathy including:

Diabetes: A majority of the cases of Neuropathy are often found in people with Diabetes, when it's referred to as Diabetic Neuropathy. This occurs when excess blood glucose injures the walls of the small blood vessels that supply nerves, particularly those in the legs (usually after a long period of time).

Heavy Alcohol Use: Most alcoholics tend to develop Peripheral Neuropathy since they often make poor choices of diet, resulting in vitamin deficiencies.

Medications: Certain medications, particularly statin drugs, which are in widespread use to combat high cholesterol, have been linked to Neuropathy. Worse, most patients who have been taking cholesterol medications have never been made aware of the link.

It has also been found that chemotherapy, which is used to treat cancer, can cause Peripheral Neuropathy.

Spinal Stenosis: Spinal stenosis is a narrowing of the spinal column that causes pressure on the spinal cord, or narrowing of the openings where spinal nerves leave the spinal column. This can lead to Peripheral Neuropathy.

Infections: Certain viral and bacterial infections including Lyme's Disease, Epstein-Barr virus, shingles (varicella-zoster), hepatitis C, diphtheria and leprosy may also cause Peripheral Neuropathy.

Trauma: Traumas like motor vehicle accidents or falls can cause damage to the peripheral nerves. Some of these traumas subsequently put too much pressure on the nerves which often goes uncorrected.

It is also possible that the process of healing from the trauma (for instance by using crutches or standing in an unnatural position for a long time) can also lead to the complication.

Treatment Options for Neuropathy

There are several classes of treatment options for Neuropathy:

Medications, therapy and home remedies.

Generally this type of treatment is aimed at helping to manage the condition(s) causing your Neuropathy since, if the underlying factor is corrected, the condition usually improves on its own.

Treatment such as medications and therapy may also help to relieve the symptoms.

Medication: There are many types of medications that have been used (wisely or otherwise) to help with the pain and other symptoms of Neuropathy including:

Anti-seizure medications: Though initially meant to be used to treat epilepsy, medications like topiramate, gabapentin, pregabalin, carbamazepine and phenytoin, have often been prescribed by doctors for nerve pain. At best this is treating the symptoms since the Peripheral Neuropathy itself remains untreated and uncorrected.

Pain relievers: Mild to moderate symptoms of the condition may be relieved by taking certain over-the-counter pain medications like non-steroidal anti-inflammatory drugs.

More-severe symptoms may be relieved by prescription painkillers as recommended by many doctors.

The obvious difficulty with taking pain medication is that it does nothing to correct the cause of the condition. As a result, the condition can be expected to worsen.

Therapies: One common therapy used to treat Neuropathy is transcutaneous electrical nerve stimulation (TENS).

It involves a therapist placing adhesive electrodes on the patient's skin and then directing a gentle electric current via the electrodes, usually at varying frequencies. If applied for about 30 minutes daily over a month, the transcutaneous electrical nerve stimulation (TENS) may help to relieve the painful symptoms.

Mechanical Vibration Therapy: This involves using vibration on the effected parts of the body. It is a simple therapy that gets results though experts are not in agreement as to how it works exactly.

The consensus is that the vibration stimulates the nerves into a growth cycle, thus reversing the Neuropathy.

Infrared Light Therapy: This is the use of infrared light to stimulate better blood flow enriched with nitric oxide to best help nerve repair which can relieve and reverse Neuropathy.

Warm Laser Therapy: This is one of the more exciting breakthroughs in the treatment of Peripheral Neuropathy.

A warm laser operating at specific wavelengths and approved by the FDA is applied to the effected areas and penetrates the tissue, reviving the nerves and causing a cycle of regeneration.

It is typical for someone suffering from Neuropathy to go through a period where they try to diagnose the condition and attempt to remedy it on their own.

When consulting with a doctor, remember to tell him or her what you have done in the past. This may help them to figure out the proper course of action for you.

Chapter 2: Diagnosing Neuropathy

The nerves that run from the spinal cord to all other parts of the body are called the peripheral nervous system and it connects the brain and the spinal cord to other body structures.

Peripheral Neuropathy is a medical condition that can be a local nerve disease, and that can also occur as a secondary manifestation of a systemic pathology.

That means that Peripheral Neuropathy can develop due to problems with other aspects of the body that, at first glance, may or may not have anything to do with the nerves.

The characteristic manifestations are paraesthesia, which is a tingling sensation, and the chronic pain of the hands or legs. Peripheral Neuropathy is relatively common in people over the age of 55. Approximately 4% of patients in this age group showed signs and symptoms of this disorder.

Causes of Peripheral Neuropathy

One of the main causes of Peripheral Neuropathy is physical trauma. Sometimes injuries cause constant pressure on the nerves. There are a great many other things that can cause it as well.

Other causes of Peripheral Neuropathy are:

- Diabetes
- Alcoholism
- HIV/SIDA
- Hepatitis
- Adverse drug reactions
- Spinal Stenosis

Peripheral Neuropathy Symptoms

A damaged nerve can cause Peripheral Neuropathy.

The manifestations are classified in: motor symptoms (having to do with the ability to move), sensory symptoms (having to do with the ability to feel) and vegetative symptoms, but often they are mixed.

The sensory symptoms are characterized by changes in the ability to feel pain, the ability to feel pressure and surfaces (tactile) and the ability to feel heat (thermal perceptions), with the appearance of:

- Paresthesias (tingling sensations)
- Inability to feel tactile stimuli such as whether or not you are touching something
- Inability to determine the joints position in space.
- Hyperaesthesia (patients can not touch even the most delicate materials due to the pain it causes).

The motor symptoms are represented by:

- Muscle weakness (not due to muscle loss)
- Muscle hypotrophy (degeneration)
- The loss of dexterity

Diagnosing Neuropathy

There are specialized investigations that can determine what the general health condition of the patient is, it may reveal the cause of the disease and it may help the doctor in making treatment plans.

The peripheral nerve recovery has a possible recovery of 2 mm a day. Depending on the evolution of the disease, on the severity of the lesion, and the time it took the patient to reach out to the specialist, the chances of recovery, in the case of this condition, are from 0 to 100%.

Diagnosing Neuropathy requires a detailed neurological exam but is fairly straightforward and does not necessarily require expensive scans.

In my office we use very tried and true methods of determining to what degree you can still feel hot/cold, tactile and other sensory perceptions. They are all simple and effective.

In diagnosing Peripheral Neuropathy, the investigation called electromyography has a very important role.

An Electromyography (EMG) followed by the Nerve Conduction Test (NCV) establishes the place where the nerve was affected and sometimes it can indicate the patient's prognosis.

An electrodiagnostic examination is a key procedure in all patients suspected of Neuropathy.

It helps certifying the presence or the absence of the sensory involvement, when this problem is only clarified by a clinical examination.

By using the electromyography, the doctor can determine if the prognosis is good. If so the patient can heal with treatment. If the lesion is definitive then recovery will be limited.

Neuropathy Treatment

The specialist treatment includes administration of various procedures. I can give you a full tour of the equipment and its effectiveness in my office.

The general goal is the recovery of motor functions of the patient as well as the ability to feel various sensations that have been lost.

The Peripheral Neuropathy treatment also includes hygiene of everyday life and some nutritional changes. For Diabetic Neuropathy a full weight loss program may be indicated.

Chapter 3: What Causes Neuropathy?

Neuropathy, also referred to as Peripheral Neuropathy, is caused by different underlying conditions. The disease damages nerves in the peripheral nervous system, brain, and spinal cord nerves but not central nervous system nerves.

Peripheral nerves are important because they carry nerve impulses from the body to the spinal cord and then to the brain. They also carry motor signals required for muscle movement from the brain to the spinal cord and then to the rest of the body.

An ordinary person cannot function normally when peripheral nerves are seriously damaged.

In fact it is dangerous to ignore.

For example, Peripheral Neuropathy may make it impossible to feel either the feet or the position of the joints in the ankles and feet.

This makes simply walking an act of faith. People report the sensation of swinging their legs forward and hoping their feet are in the right place to catch them - with each step.

It is also possible to seriously damage the feet by stepping on sharp objects but not being able to feel it.

There are reports of people discovering nails through their feet hours after the walk they took as well as other serious injuries.

Patients of Peripheral Neuropathy also report feelings of abnormal sensations that commonly occur in the feet.

The three main types of nerves involved on Peripheral Neuropathy are autonomic nerves, motor nerves, and sensory nerves.

Autonomic nerves regulate the automatic functions of the body.

Such functions include the heart rate, sweating, and the production of hormones among others that are carried out by the body automatically.

The conscious control of muscles is achieved through motor nerves. Sensations of heat and cold and even the position of joints are communicated to the brain through sensory nerves.

Common Causes of Neuropathy

Causes of Peripheral Neuropathy can be classified as physical trauma, genetic, repetitive injury, infection, metabolic problems, drugs, or toxins. Take a closer look at some of the causes and its effects:

Diabetes: A common cause of Neuropathy is Diabetes, which is metabolic disorder.

Persons suffering from Diabetes suffer injuries on the walls of blood vessels that supply blood to the nerves.

As a result, patients are unable to feel pain due to nerve damage. This type of nerve damage is common in the legs. In the US, half of diabetic patients suffer from Diabetic Neuropathy.

Pressure on the Nerves: Nerve pressure also causes Neuropathy. Accidents that cause traumatic injuries result in pressure on the nerves.

Other conditions that cause Peripheral Neuropathy include liver and kidney diseases, HIV/AIDS, too much alcohol intake over many years, nutritional deficiencies, cancer, diphtheria, among other diseases and conditions.

Drugs that produce Neuropathy include some cardiac drugs, blood pressure drugs, some cancer drugs, psychiatric drugs, anti-seizure drugs, dermatitis treatment, anti-hypertensive drugs, cholesterol drugs and alcoholism treatment drugs.

Notice that this is quite a list and covers a wide range of medical conditions.

Each cause described above created conditions that lead to the damage of the peripheral nerves thereby causing Neuropathy.

The nerves may be starved of blood supply, inflamed, or undergo damage due to too much pressure.

For example, systemic diseases cause Neuropathy by affecting the body's ability to transform nutrients into forms required for use by the body.

In addition, when toxins accumulate in the body due to liver and kidney disorders, they damage the nerves.

Most kidney failure patients require dialysis and eventually develop Neuropathy. Hormonal imbalances cause Neuropathy by interfering with metabolic process and removal of body fluids causing too much pressure on the nerves leading to damage.

You can see that are there quite a number of ways that a person could wind up with Neuropathy. That is precisely why it is so prevalent today.

Serious cases of Peripheral Neuropathy are life threatening and patients with symptoms consistent with those associated with the disease should schedule a consultation with a practitioner who is able to get results.

If you are in Southern California, my contact information is at the end of this book.

The underlying cause of the condition needs to be identified and treatment administered. An untreated condition leads to loss of nerve function, paralysis, muscle wasting, gangrene, and serious infection.

Because Diabetes is commonly associated with the condition, proper management of the Diabetes is critical.

Data from around the USA indicates that Neuropathy is the common cause of foot problems and ulcers. Managing Peripheral Neuropathy therefore lessens some complications associated with Diabetes.

Chapter 4: Different Types of Neuropathy

Neuropathy is generally associated with damage of the nerves specifically in the peripheral nervous system. The nerves that are outside the spinal cord and the brain are damaged; however, the central nervous system is not affected. Neuropathy is caused by exposure to toxins, physical trauma, infections, metabolic problems and repetitive injury.

Three types of Neuropathy are Diabetic Neuropathy, Peripheral Neuropathy, and Cranial Neuropathy.

Diabetic Neuropathy

This condition involves damage of the nerve cells in diabetic patients. The damage is usually as a result of high blood sugar over a long period of time which eventually compromises many aspects of health. Among those are the nerves.

Diabetic Neuropathy usually affects the nerve fibers in the feet and legs. However, the condition could also be found affecting other parts of the body and presents with symptoms such as numbness, pain, problems in urinary tract system, digestive system, heart and the blood vessels.

Diabetic Neuropathy can be prevented by doing what it takes to keep your blood sugar under control and living a healthy lifestyle.

<u>Peripheral Neuropathy</u>

This condition mainly affects sensory nerves, motor nerves, and autonomic nerves.

As a result, the muscle movement, body sensations, and various control functions are affected.

Beginning stages of Peripheral Neuropathy starts from the longest nerves that create symptoms that include a burning pain, dizziness that results from changes in blood pressure, muscle weakness (especially when motor nerves are affected), poor coordination, high touch sensitivity, digestive problems (resulting from affected autonomic nerves), and sharp electric pain.

Individuals experiencing unusual tingling, pain and weakness of their hands should not delay seeking medical help to avoid further damage to the peripheral nerve.

Cranial Neuropathy

Cranial Neuropathy consists of damaged nerves surrounding the skull and the cranium.

These nerves control functions such as hearing, vision, facial movement and other organ's actions. In most cases, Cranial Neuropathy is a secondary condition that results from other medical conditions such as Diabetes.

Cranial Neuropathy may be caused by conditions such as Sarcoidosis, Lyme's Disease and HIV infection. The symptoms of Cranial Neuropathy may clear after some months but may be permanent in some cases.

The symptoms in this condition vary significantly depending on the nerves affected.

In most cases, one of the most common damages occurs in the facial nerve which results in facial pain and eye muscle paralysis. Additionally, this condition has other complications such as twitches, Bell's Palsy, and facial tics.

Treatment of the conditions may range from treating the cause, to use of anti-inflammatory drugs and use of eye ointments among others.

Autonomic Neuropathy

Autonomic Neuropathy is a nerve disorder caused by autoimmune diseases, amyloidosis (abnormal protein buildup), Parkinson's Disease, nerve injury, hereditary disorders and some types of drugs used in the treatment of cancer i.e. chemotherapy.

It affects the parts of the body that are not under your conscious control such as the heart rate, digestion, perspiration and blood pressure.

Although it is not known as a specific disease, it is often referred or associated with damage to autonomic nerves.

The different types of Neuropathy described should be verified with your chosen physician. For a complete diagnosis, please contact a physician to get started towards maintaining and keeping great health. The overall results are priceless!

Chapter 5: Neuropathy Symptoms

People suffering from Neuropathy report feeling a tingling or burning sensation at the onset of the disease.

This sensation is similar to the sensation felt when one wears a thin stocking or glove.

Neuropathy symptoms depend on the type of Neuropathy and type of nerves affected. The nerves that reach the toes are affected first because the condition affects the longest nerves first.

Sensory nerve damage has the following symptoms:

- Numbness or tingling sensation in the feet/ hands
- Burning pains
- Sharp pains
- Acute sensitivity to touch
- Noticeable changes on the skin, nail, or hair

- Poor coordination

Neuropathy Symptoms

Symptoms of Neuropathy of the motor nerves may include

- Muscle weakness
- Complete paralysis

Typical symptoms of Autonomic Nerve Neuropathy are:

- Heat intolerance
- Digestive problems
- Dizziness caused by changes in blood pressure

Diabetic patients suffering from Diabetic Neuropathy are often asymptomatic. However, healthcare professionals can identify slight tell-tale signs of the condition in the form of reduced ankle reflexes and painless foot injuries.

Patients report pain in the toes, feet, or legs that can be either "stabbing" or "burning".

This pain is severe and troublesome at night leading to loss of sleep or troubled sleep.

Smaller nerves produce burning like pain while larger ones produce electric tingling sensation.

Symptoms of Diabetic Neuropathy are distinguishable through the types of nerves involved.

Diabetic Neuropathy caused by autonomic nerves produce the following symptoms:

- Abnormal heart effects such as heart beating too fast or Tachycardia
- Urinary problems
- Sexual problems
- Low blood pressure when standing up

Physicians look out for following Diabetic Neuropathy symptoms:

- Reduced ankle reflexes
- Infections
- Gangrene
- Painless injuries

Persons exhibiting these symptoms should immediately consult a doctor for medical check-up. Because Diabetic Neuropathy is common with diabetic patients, regular examination of the disease is advisable during the course of Diabetes management as the condition is asymptomatic.

Chapter 6: Managing and Treating Neuropathy Symptoms

For diabetics and those suffering from the debilitating effects of other diseases and health conditions, (e.g., kidney and liver disease, cancer, Lyme's Disease, etc.), Neuropathy is one of the most vexing and difficult complications to treat and manage.

Defined as nerve damage in the peripheral nervous system, symptoms normally begin with a tingling or burning sensation in the feet and hands, which often spreads to the legs and arms. More severe symptoms include pain, muscle weakness or paralysis, blood pressure issues, and heart, digestive or sexual problems.

While there is no universal cure for Neuropathy, there are a variety of non-invasive, effective treatments to help manage pain and improve function:

Transcutaneous Electrical Nerve Stimulation (TENS)

In this form of treatment, electrodes are attached to the skin using an adhesive and a gentle current is delivered to the affected areas at varying frequencies.

TENS is normally performed daily for a half hour over a period of 30 days, with some patients reporting pain relief and increased feeling and sensation from the therapy.

Massage Therapy

For many with Diabetes or chemotherapy-induced Neuropathy massage therapy has been shown to be one of the most effective ways to manage and reduce pain, and the protocol used by massage therapists is an excellent way to monitor symptoms.

The protocol begins with examining the feet, looking for sores, redness, cracks in the skin, toenail fungus (common on cancer patients) and dark spots (gas gangrene first appears in this form).

Therapists then begin with light pressure, charting the patient's pain response, working from the feet or hands up to the ankle, legs, wrists and arms.

Performed once a week, massage therapy can also help restore range of motion, improve circulation and stimulate nerves, and the self-massage techniques that many therapists teach patients can lead to improvement as well.

<u>Physical Therapy</u>

PT doesn't cure Neuropathy, although there are instances in which physical therapists have been able to eliminate entrapment Neuropathy by freeing the trapped nerve.

It can help with muscle weakness or atrophy, though, and it can also improve strength, balance, coordination and flexibility.

Topical Creams

The advantage of these kinds of creams is that they can be applied directly to the pain site, where they act as local anesthetics, numbing the site to provide relief.

Many of these products contain capsaicin, a painkiller derived from chili peppers, while others use botanical oils.

There is also a medical grade topical cream available from my office which relies on a menthol base and is very effective.

Neuropathy Support Supplements

This is a broad category that includes both supplements as well as holistic and dietary approaches to managing Neuropathy.

The most common is a formula that combines alpha lipoic acid, benfotiamine and methylcobalamine in a single, natural herbal product.

Other promising possibilities include B12 shots (which can actually cure Neuropathy if it is caused by a severe B12 deficiency), acetyl-L-carnitine, and gamma linolenic acid.

Herbal approaches include curcumin, geranium oil, evening primrose oil, and fish oil supplements with omega-3 fatty acids.

In a later chapter I outline more of the helpful vitamins and herbs in more detail.

The nutritional approach seems most effective when combined with other treatments.

Mechanical and Vertical Sound Vibration

This is yet another broad category that includes several innovative approaches.

There is some evidence that applying low-level mechanical or electrical noise to the skin of healthy subjects and older adults can significantly enhance tactile sensitivity.

Stimulation is applied to the foot, being careful to establish and observe a sensitivity threshold.

The mechanisms behind improvement aren't fully understood, but this kind of noise may add mechanical energy that enhances vibration transmission through the dermal tissue.

It may also change the so-called "pain gate" in the spinal cord to help with nerve function and restore tactile sensitivity.

Sound vibration is an analogous technique that has also been effective treating auditory

Neuropathy, which occurs when sound enters the inner ear but signals from the inner ear to the brain are impaired due to damage to inner hair cells.

The treatment involves standing on a vibrating platform, which activates body's stretch reflex for spontaneous muscle contraction, with the rest allowing the body to recover enough to sometimes restore function.

I use both of these techniques in my office to good effect.

Infrared Light Therapy

Light therapy using infrared LEDs has been effective as a general treatment across the spectrum of different types of Neuropathy and symptoms.

An LED light "boot" or blanket is used on the effected areas and stimulates the blood circulation. This releases nitric oxide which in turn aids in the healing of the nerves.

Laser Therapy

One of the most recent breakthroughs in the treatment of Neuropathy is the use of a specially designed warm laser.

I have found this to be the most effective of the various treatments.

These warm laser medical devices are FDA approved and are used on the surface of the skin. The special laser light stimulates the deep tissue and provides both relief from pain and stimulates healing.

Chapter 7: Natural Options for Handling the Symptoms of Neuropathy

According to a report released by the Neuropathy Association an estimated 20 million individuals suffer from mild to severe forms of Neuropathy.

This painful and debilitating condition can significantly decrease a patient's quality of life and can result in serious complications including foot ulcers, cardiac arrhythmias, and death.

There are numerous medications that are used to control the symptoms of Neuropathy, but there are also natural supplements that have been proven to reduce the symptoms without the side effects associated with many medications.

Benfotiamine

Benfotiamine is a man-made form of vitamin B1.

It is also known as thiamine, a vitamin that is essential for nerves to function properly.

Taking a vitamin B1 supplement ensures that the body has adequate levels of B1 in it which can result in a decrease in the symptoms of Neuropathy.

It has been shown to be particularly effective in decreasing pain associated with Diabetic Neuropathy and it also reduces microvascular damage that results from frequent high blood sugar levels.

Vitamin B2

Vitamin B2 (also known as riboflavin) is an antioxidant that works to make certain the nervous system is properly functioning and fights off free radicals in the body that cause pain.

Physicians have found that having a deficient amount of vitamin B2 can lead to or worsen the symptoms of Peripheral Neuropathy. This vitamin is easily obtained.

Vitamin B6

Vitamin B6 (commonly called pyridoxone), is an

essential vitamin that is required in sufficient levels for fat, carbohydrate, and protein metabolism.

Deficient levels in the body can result in fatigue, moodiness, irritability, and Neuropathy.

Researchers have found that almost all diabetics suffering from Neuropathy have a vitamin B6 deficiency resulting in worsening symptoms.

As a result supplementation provides the amount the body requires and symptoms of Neuropathy decrease.

<u>Vitamin B12</u>

Vitamin B12 (also referred to as methylcobalamine) is necessary to protect the body against neurological diseases.

High levels of methylcobalamine have been proven to regenerate neurons and the myelin sheath that provides protection for the nerve axons and peripheral nerves.

Patients that have received injections of vitamin B12 in the form of methylcobalamine have reported decreased Neuropathy symptoms as well as improved balance and less weakness.

Vitamin D

Vitamin D promotes nerve and neuron growth. Deficient levels of Vitamin D have been determined to impair pain receptor function, increase the potential for nerve damage, and to be a risk factor for Diabetic Neuropathy.

Recent research has found that Vitamin D supplementation can slow down progression of the condition and significantly decreases the amount of neuropathic pain felt.

Vitamin D is usually accompanied by Vitamin A.

R-Alpha Lipoic Acid

R-Alpha Lipoic Acid is an antioxidant produced by the body and found in all cells.

Studies have shown that its effectiveness at killing free radicals proves beneficial to patients suffering from Peripheral Neuropathy.

Patients who have received this in IV form report decreased burning, tingling, itching, and numbness associated with nerve damage.

It has also decreased symptoms associated with autonomic Neuropathy when taken orally.

The gold standard for alpha lipoic acid treatment is a time released formula, which will provide a constant supply of alpha lipoic acid for the nerves. Most ALA supplements DO NOT contain time released ALA because of the increased cost.

Natural Herbs

There are also numerous herbs available that have proven to be beneficial in the reduction of Neuropathy symptoms.

Feverfew Extract has been found to help control the symptoms of Neuropathy, specifically nerve pain.

Oat Straw Extract acts to decrease general pain, nerve pain, and helps sooth the itchy skin that some patients develop with Neuropathy.

Skullcap Extract works to cause a tranquilizing effect on the nervous system.

It has a tremendous impact on decreasing Neuropathy symptoms including pain and tingling.

Finally, Flower Passion is an herb that has been found to eliminate symptoms especially nerve pain. Many patients take more than one supplement for maximum relief.

Before beginning any supplements it is essential to speak with your physician to find out if there may be any possible interactions with your current medicine regimen and to determine what dosages are appropriate for you.

Be aware that most patients report it takes approximately three weeks to begin seeing the benefits associated with taking these supplements.

Chapter 8: Neuropathy Avoidance and Reversing Neuropathy

Neuropathy is a complication which is found in a number of different underlying conditions.

It is damage to the nerves which are outside the central nervous system.

As such it is usually referred to as Peripheral Neuropathy since the nerves it affects are found in the peripheral nervous system.

It is also sometimes referred to as Polyneuropathy because it typically affects multiple nerves simultaneously.

When no underlying cause has been diagnosed, it is referred to as Idiopathic Neuropathy.

As covered earlier, there are a number of factors which lead to Neuropathy including physical trauma, repetitive injury, metabolic problems, and exposure to infections and toxins.

Others are medical conditions such as Diabetes, HIV/AIDS, kidney disease, lymphoma, multiple myeloma, diphtheria and Guillain-Barré syndrome.

Neuropathy affects sensory nerves, motor nerves and involuntary nerves.

Neuropathy Avoidance

Avoiding Neuropathy entails taking measures which limit the conditions which lead to its occurrence. Some of the measures are the following:

Taking care when participating in sports or performing any physical activity.

Any direct injury to a nerve can lead to the emergence of Neuropathy.

Therefore special care should be taken in terms of using protective gear to avoid or mitigate injury.

<u>Treating predisposing medical conditions.</u>

Treating diseases such as Diabetes, kidney disease and the other conditions mentioned earlier.

Patients with these conditions need vigilant treatment and monitoring in order to prevent those conditions from degeneration into Neuropathy.

Taking precaution against getting exposed to toxins or viral infection:

Precautions against toxins include poisons and dysfunctional medicines. The precaution can take the form of avoiding exposure and prompt management in case exposure takes place. Avoid placing repeated pressure on a nerve.

Take daily vitamins to help strengthen the immune system:

Vitamin B-12 in particular is critical in the prevention of Neuropathy. This can be done through eating foods which are rich in Vitamin B-12 or taking Vitamin B-12 supplements.

Reversing Neuropathy

"Reversing" Neuropathy entails taking actions which can reverse the negative effects of Neuropathy. Medically this involves taking steps to eradicate symptoms only.

Yes, that's correct, in medical circles it is typically considered reversed when the symptoms abate. To that end you can expect to be treated with drugs.

Prosthetic Pain: Prosthetic pain can be mitigated using drugs which can mitigate the pain. Such drugs typically include pain killers or pain relief therapies.

The drugs must be prescribed by a doctor for a specific patient; but the common drugs are brand names such as Oxecta, Oxycotin and Cozip. Skin patches containing anesthetics can also be used to relieve the pain.

I am not in favor of drug treatments to handle symptoms. In my office we go for a true reversal, which would be the re-growth of the damaged nerves themselves where possible.

Non Drug Measures: Non-drug measures include wearing garments which can cause minimal irritation, covering sensitive areas with wound dressing and using cold packs. Such measures are useful for minimizing the discomfort that is results from the condition.

Various Therapies: Other complementary therapies such as stress-relief, meditation, massage, vitamin therapy and relaxation techniques can be used alongside regular treatment. Such measures will boost a patient's ability to cope with the condition.

Specified Treatment: There are also treatments which are targeted towards strains of Neuropathy which are caused by specific conditions such as Diabetes.

This involves treating the specific ailments such as urinary symptoms, digestive problems, sexual dysfunctions and orthostatic hypotension.

Overall, given the fact that Neuropathy is caused by multiple factors, mitigating and treating it requires multi-faceted approach.

The approaches that are listed are useful for both avoiding and reversing Neuropathy. With the help of a licensed physician that specializes in this area, help is available.

Chapter 9: Neuropathy and Lifestyle

Changes to Make to Reduce or Eliminate Neuropathy Pain and Symptoms

Living with pain everyday is not only uncomfortable, but depressing as well. One common cause for ongoing pain is the condition known as Neuropathy. There are various diseases, which cause painful nerve damage in the human body.

In fact, the medical industry has identified 100 known types of nerve pain. In America today, about 3% of the population suffers from some form of nerve pain and its symptoms. Symptoms include numbness or tingling in the extremities, the degree of which can range from moderate to severe.

The sufferer may experience painful pins and needles sensations in the feet or hands and fingers.

Feelings of intense heat or cold due to decreased circulation in the limbs are other symptoms. Ongoing nerve pain is the basis for diagnosing patients with Neuropathy.

The pain and symptoms of Neuropathy can affect one's ability to go about functioning normally in their everyday life.

However, making a few simple lifestyle changes can limit the risk of one's health from spiraling down, due to the pain of living with damaged nerves that can lead to inactivity.

The less active the person is, the more chances chronic pain has to restrict mobility.

The last thing the patient wants is to become bed ridden, so the faster one can make lifestyle changes to reduce or eliminate Neuropathy pain and symptoms, the better chances they have for maintaining a happy and productive life.

Change Your Diet

People living with Neuropathy and its symptoms should begin by changing their diet.

One of the most important diet changes to make is to include more fruits and vegetables. In fact, one should switch over to diet heavy in vegetables.

Eat lots of green leafy vegetables. Be sure to add more of the darker fruits such as blueberries and pomegranates, purple grapes and black plumbs to the diet.

This ensures the body gets enough of the vitamins, minerals and antioxidants it needs to support health and energy levels.

<u>Stop Smoking</u>

<u>Stop the Consumption of Alcohol</u>

<u>Add an Exercise Routine</u>

Exercising is very important. It helps keep the body limber and the muscles strong. Before beginning, take the time to learn how to exercise properly to avoid injury and do not forget to do a warm up before exercising and a cool down afterward.

Get at least two 15 minutes sessions of moderate exercise in each day. Low impact exercises are best, such as walking and swimming.

Wear Loose Clothing and Shoes

Tight socks and shoes can cause poor circulation in the feet and legs. Wear loose-fitting clothes to help reduce pain and symptoms.

Wear the proper footwear that your doctor recommends for people who have Neuropathy pain in the feet.

Eating right, exercising the right way, and wearing the right type of clothing, are important lifestyle changes to make to reduce or eliminate Neuropathy pain and symptoms.

Testimonials

When I first came to the clinic, I could barely walk. Now I can do almost anything: exercising, and dancing... I really recommend Dr. Hashimoto, he is a wonderful doctor.

-Vicki

When I came here, my hands were numb and I had a headache every day. Since that time, my hands are no longer numb and my headaches are gone!

-Marla D.

I am very happy that I am able to walk, because I was not able to walk when I first came in to see Dr. Hashimoto. Now, believe it or not, I am walking without a cane!

-Maria H.

I have been coming to Dr. Hashimoto for almost 2 months because of pain and trouble sleeping. Thanks to Dr. Naota I am no longer in pain, I sleep better, and I can dance now!

-Lernal

Since I have been coming to see Dr. Hashimoto, the pain and numbness in my toes and feet have much improved.

-Jennifer

When I first came to Dr. Hashimoto, I could hardly walk with a cane. Now, I'm ready to go tap dancing and mountain climbing! I really appreciate it!

-Bob

I just finished my first treatment, and I am able to walk. When I first came in here today, I was limping. Now, I have lost my limp.

-Betty

I can walk much better and I feel much better. He has taken very good care of me. Thank you.

-Barbara T.

PERIPHERAL
NEUROPATHY
101:

A GUIDE FOR PATIENTS

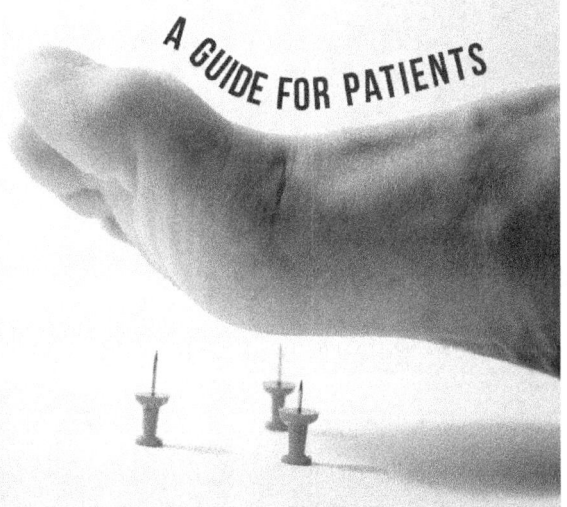

DR. HASHIMOTO

Table of Contents

Introduction To The Easy-To Read Section

The following is a reprint of the book, *A Doctor's Guide To Peripheral Neuropathy*.

This book is two books in one, or rather, it is one book printed twice.

The first (approx.) half is the book printed with normal lay-out conventions which makes it the easiest way for many people to read the book.

Peripheral Neuropathy, as you will learn, afflicts a wide range of people. A good many have their best eyesight behind them. To address this we have changed the lay-out and have adopted larger print and formatting rules that are the latest in easy to read type.

The book has then been reprinted and reformatted with large easy to read type and with font selection, spacing and other formatting specifically designed to allow the reader, who would normally have trouble reading "normal" printed text, to read comfortably and easily.

Chapter 1: What is Neuropathy?

Neuropathy is a condition in which a person experiences pain and numbness often in the hands and feet, though it may occur in other parts of the body as well.

The word itself betrays the general and somewhat mysterious nature of the disease. Neuro- of or related to nerves and –pathy a disease or ailment of.

In medical circles, one can see that a lot of different conditions could be attributed to "something wrong with the nerves".

Regardless of the vague definition, Peripheral Neuropathy sometimes referred to as Polyneuropathy, is typically diagnosed when a person has pain or numbness where there is no direct or observable cause for it.

The complication occurs as a result of nerve damage in the peripheral nervous system. There are 3 main types of nerves that can be involved:

Autonomic nerves: These regulate heart rate, sweating, blood pressure and other automatic functions of the body.

Motor nerves: Control the body muscles and are usually under conscious control.

Sensory nerves: These transmit sensations (such as information about heat and cold) from other body parts to the brain.

Symptoms of Neuropathy

Most people with Neuropathy often report feeling a tingling pain or burning sensation. This is most commonly in the feet.

Generally, an individual's specific symptoms may depend on the kind of nerves affected.

Common symptoms and signs of Neuropathy include:

- Numbness and tingling sensation in, usually, the hands or feet but which can spread to the arms and legs. This sensation can make sleep very difficult.

- Sharp, electric-like pain.

- The sense that one is stepping off into nothing with each step.

- Burning pain where no burn has occurred. Often it is impossible to point to an exact source of the pain as it will seem to be in an entire area such as the whole foot.

- Muscle weakness /paralysis.

- Heat intolerance. Running one's hands under warm water may cause discomfort

- High sensitivity to touch. Even light brushes may prove to be very uncomfortable.

- Dizziness due to changes in the blood pressure. This often shows up when standing up after sitting for some time.

Causes of Neuropathy

Since the complication may be caused by different factors or a combination of factors, it is not easy to pinpoint its exact cause(s).

This fact is well known to many Neuropathy sufferers as they have often tried many different treatments.

There are certain factors, however, that are associated with development of Neuropathy including:

Diabetes: A majority of the cases of Neuropathy are often found in people with Diabetes, when it's referred to as Diabetic Neuropathy. This occurs when excess blood glucose injures the walls of the small blood vessels that supply nerves, particularly those in the legs (usually after a long period of time).

Heavy Alcohol Use: Most alcoholics tend to develop Peripheral Neuropathy since they often make poor choices of diet, resulting in vitamin deficiencies.

Medications: Certain medications, particularly statin drugs, which are in widespread use to combat high cholesterol, have been linked to Neuropathy. Worse, most patients who have been taking cholesterol medications have never been made aware of the link.

It has also been found that chemotherapy, which is used to treat cancer, can cause Peripheral Neuropathy.

Spinal Stenosis: Spinal stenosis is a narrowing of the spinal column that causes pressure on the spinal cord, or narrowing of the openings where spinal nerves leave the spinal column.

This can lead to Peripheral Neuropathy.

Infections: Certain viral and bacterial infections including Lyme's Disease, Epstein-Barr virus, shingles (varicella-zoster), hepatitis C, diphtheria and leprosy may also cause Peripheral Neuropathy.

Trauma: Traumas like motor vehicle accidents or falls can cause damage to the peripheral nerves. Some of these traumas subsequently put too much pressure on the nerves which often goes uncorrected.

It is also possible that the process of healing from the trauma (for instance by using crutches or standing in an unnatural position for a long time) can also lead to the complication.

Treatment Options for Neuropathy

There are several classes of treatment options for Neuropathy:

Medications, therapy and home remedies.

Generally this type of treatment is aimed at helping to manage the condition(s) causing your Neuropathy since, if the underlying factor is corrected, the condition usually improves on its own.

Treatment such as medications and therapy may also help to relieve the symptoms.

Medication: There are many types of medications that have been used (wisely or otherwise) to help with the pain and other symptoms of Neuropathy including:

Anti-seizure medications: Though initially meant to be used to treat epilepsy, medications like topiramate, gabapentin, pregabalin, carbamazepine and phenytoin, have often been prescribed by doctors for nerve pain. At best this is treating the symptoms since the Peripheral Neuropathy itself remains untreated and uncorrected.

Pain relievers: Mild to moderate symptoms of the condition may be relieved by taking certain over-the-counter pain medications like non-steroidal anti-inflammatory drugs. More-severe symptoms may be relieved by prescription painkillers as recommended by many doctors.

The obvious difficulty with taking pain medication is that it does nothing to correct the cause of the condition. As a result, the condition can be expected to worsen.

Therapies: One common therapy used to treat Neuropathy is transcutaneous electrical nerve stimulation (TENS).

It involves a therapist placing adhesive electrodes on the patient's skin and then directing a gentle electric current via the electrodes, usually at varying frequencies. If applied for about 30 minutes daily over a month, the transcutaneous electrical nerve stimulation (TENS) may help to relieve the painful symptoms.

Mechanical Vibration Therapy: This involves using vibration on the effected parts of the body. It is a simple therapy that gets results though experts are not in agreement as to how it works exactly. The consensus is that the vibration stimulates the nerves into a growth cycle, thus reversing the Neuropathy.

Infrared Light Therapy: This is the use of infrared light to stimulate better blood flow enriched with nitric oxide to best help nerve repair which can relieve and reverse Neuropathy.

Warm Laser Therapy: This is one of the more exciting breakthroughs in the treatment of Peripheral Neuropathy.

A warm laser operating at specific wavelengths and approved by the FDA is applied to the effected areas and penetrates the tissue, reviving the nerves and causing a cycle of regeneration.

It is typical for someone suffering from Neuropathy to go through a period where they try to diagnose the condition and attempt to remedy it on their own.

When consulting with a doctor, remember to tell him or her what you have done in the past. This may help them to figure out the proper course of action for you.

Chapter 2: Diagnosing Neuropathy

The nerves that run from the spinal cord to all other parts of the body are called the peripheral nervous system and it connects the brain and the spinal cord to other body structures.

Peripheral Neuropathy is a medical condition that can be a local nerve disease, and that can also occur as a secondary manifestation of a systemic pathology.

That means that Peripheral Neuropathy can develop due to problems with other aspects of the body that, at first glance, may or may not have anything to do with the nerves.

The characteristic manifestations are paraesthesia, which is a tingling sensation, and the chronic pain of the hands or legs.

Peripheral Neuropathy is relatively common in people over the age of 55. Approximately 4% of patients in this age group showed signs and symptoms of this disorder.

Causes of Peripheral Neuropathy

One of the main causes of Peripheral Neuropathy is physical trauma. Sometimes injuries cause constant pressure on the nerves. There are a great many other things that can cause it as well.

Other causes of Peripheral Neuropathy are:

- Diabetes
- Alcoholism
- HIV/SIDA
- Hepatitis
- Adverse drug reactions
- Spinal Stenosis

Peripheral Neuropathy Symptoms

A damaged nerve can cause Peripheral Neuropathy. The manifestations are classified in: motor symptoms (having to do with the ability to move), sensory symptoms (having to do with the ability to feel) and vegetative symptoms, but often they are mixed.

The sensory symptoms are characterized by changes in the ability to feel pain, the ability to feel pressure and surfaces (tactile) and the ability to feel heat (thermal perceptions), with the appearance of:

- Paresthesias (tingling sensations)
- Inability to feel tactile stimuli such as whether or not you are touching something

- Inability to determine the joints position in space.

- Hyperaesthesia (patients can not touch even the most delicate materials due to the pain it causes).

The motor symptoms are represented by:

- Muscle weakness (not due to muscle loss)

- Muscle hypotrophy (degeneration)

- The loss of dexterity

Diagnosing Neuropathy

There are specialized investigations that can determine what the general health condition of the patient is, it may reveal the cause of the disease and it may help the doctor in making treatment plans.

The peripheral nerve recovery has a possible recovery of 2 mm a day. Depending on the evolution of the disease, on the severity of the lesion, and the time it took the patient to reach out to the specialist, the chances of recovery, in the case of this condition, are from 0 to 100%.

Diagnosing Neuropathy requires a detailed neurological exam but is fairly straightforward and does not necessarily require expensive scans.

In my office we use very tried and true methods of determining to what degree you can still feel hot/cold, tactile and other sensory perceptions. They are all simple and effective.

In diagnosing Peripheral Neuropathy, the investigation called electromyography has a very important role.

An Electromyography (EMG) followed by the Nerve Conduction Test (NCV) establishes the place where the nerve was affected and sometimes it can indicate the patient's prognosis.

An electrodiagnostic examination is a key procedure in all patients suspected of Neuropathy.

It helps certifying the presence or the absence of the sensory involvement, when this problem is only clarified by a clinical examination.

By using the electromyography, the doctor can determine if the prognosis is good. If so the patient can heal with treatment. If the lesion is definitive then recovery will be limited.

Neuropathy Treatment

The specialist treatment includes the administration of various procedures done in house. I can give you a full tour of the equipment and its effectiveness in my office.

The general goal is the recovery of motor functions of the patient as well as the ability to feel various sensations that have been lost.

The Peripheral Neuropathy treatment also includes hygiene of everyday life and some nutritional changes.

For Diabetic Neuropathy a full weight loss program may be indicated.

Chapter 3: What Causes Neuropathy?

Neuropathy, also referred to as Peripheral Neuropathy, is caused by different underlying conditions. The disease damages nerves in the peripheral nervous system, brain, and spinal cord nerves but not central nervous system nerves.

Peripheral nerves are important because they carry nerve impulses from the body to the spinal cord and then to the brain.

They also carry motor signals required for muscle movement from the brain to the spinal cord and then to the rest of the body.

An ordinary person cannot function normally when peripheral nerves are seriously damaged.

For example, Peripheral Neuropathy may make it impossible to feel either the feet or the position of the joints in the ankles and feet.

This makes simply walking an act of faith. People report the sensation of

swinging their legs forward and hoping their feet are in the right place to catch them - with each step.

It is also possible to seriously damage the feet by stepping on sharp objects but not being able to feel it.

There are reports of people discovering nails through their feet hours after the walk they took as well as other serious injuries.

Patients of Peripheral Neuropathy also report feelings of abnormal sensations that commonly occur in the feet.

The three main types of nerves involved on Peripheral Neuropathy are

autonomic nerves, motor nerves, and sensory nerves.

Autonomic nerves regulate the automatic functions of the body. Such functions include the heart rate, sweating, and the production of hormones among others that are carried out by the body automatically.

The conscious control of muscles is achieved through motor nerves. Sensations of heat and cold and even the position of joints are communicated to the brain through sensory nerves.

Common Causes of Neuropathy

Causes of Peripheral Neuropathy can

be classified as physical trauma, genetic, repetitive injury, infection, metabolic problems, drugs, or toxins. Take a closer look at some of the causes and its effects:

Diabetes: A common cause of Neuropathy is Diabetes, which is metabolic disorder.

Persons suffering from Diabetes suffer injuries on the walls of blood vessels that supply blood to the nerves.

As a result, patients are unable to feel pain due to nerve damage. This type of nerve damage is common in the legs. In the US, half of diabetic patients suffer from Diabetic Neuropathy.

Pressure on the Nerves: Nerve pressure also causes Neuropathy. Accidents that cause traumatic injuries result in pressure on the nerves.

Other conditions that cause Peripheral Neuropathy include liver and kidney diseases, HIV/AIDS, too much alcohol intake over many years, nutritional deficiencies, cancer, diphtheria, among other diseases and conditions.

Drugs that produce Neuropathy include some cardiac drugs, blood pressure drugs, some cancer drugs, psychiatric drugs, anti-seizure drugs, dermatitis treatment, anti-hypertensive drugs, cholesterol drugs and alcoholism treatment drugs.

Notice that this is quite a list and covers a wide range of medical conditions.

Each cause described above created conditions that lead to the damage of the peripheral nerves thereby causing Neuropathy.

The nerves may be starved of blood supply, inflamed, or undergo damage due to too much pressure. For example, systemic diseases cause Neuropathy by affecting the body's ability to transform nutrients into forms required for use by the body.

In addition, when toxins accumulate in the body due to liver and kidney disorders, they damage the nerves.

Most kidney failure patients require dialysis and eventually develop Neuropathy. Hormonal imbalances cause Neuropathy by interfering with metabolic process and removal of body fluids causing too much pressure on the nerves leading to damage.

You can see that are there quite a number of ways that a person could wind up with Neuropathy. That is precisely why it is so prevalent today.

Serious cases of Peripheral Neuropathy are life threatening and patients with symptoms consistent with those associated with the disease should schedule a consultation with a practitioner who is able to get results. If you are in Southern California, my contact information is at the end of this book.

The underlying cause of the condition needs to be identified and treatment administered. An untreated condition leads to loss of nerve function, paralysis, muscle wasting, gangrene, and serious infection.

Because Diabetes is commonly associated with the condition, proper management of the Diabetes is critical.

Data from around the USA indicates that Neuropathy is the common cause of foot problems and ulcers.

Managing Peripheral Neuropathy therefore lessens some complications associated with Diabetes.

Chapter 4: Different Types of Neuropathy

Neuropathy is generally associated with damage of the nerves specifically in the peripheral nervous system. The nerves that are outside the spinal cord and the brain are damaged; however, the central nervous system is not affected. Neuropathy is caused by exposure to toxins, physical trauma, infections, metabolic problems and repetitive injury.

Three types of Neuropathy are Diabetic Neuropathy, Peripheral Neuropathy, and Cranial Neuropathy.

Diabetic Neuropathy

This condition involves damage of the nerve cells in diabetic patients.

The damage is usually as a result of high blood sugar over a long period of time which eventually compromises many aspects of health. Among those are the nerves.

Diabetic Neuropathy usually affects the nerve fibers in the feet and legs. However, the condition could also be found affecting other parts of the body and presents with symptoms such as numbness, pain, problems in urinary tract system, digestive system, heart and the blood vessels.

Diabetic Neuropathy can be prevented by doing what it takes to keep your blood sugar under control and living a healthy lifestyle.

Peripheral Neuropathy

This condition mainly affects sensory nerves, motor nerves, and autonomic nerves.

As a result, the muscle movement, body sensations, and various control functions are affected.

Beginning stages of Peripheral Neuropathy starts from the longest nerves that create symptoms that include a burning pain, dizziness that results from changes in blood pressure, muscle weakness (especially when motor nerves are affected), poor coordination, high touch sensitivity, digestive problems (resulting from affected autonomic nerves), and sharp electric pain.

Individuals experiencing unusual tingling, pain and weakness of their hands should not delay seeking medical help to avoid further damage to the peripheral nerve.

Cranial Neuropathy

Cranial Neuropathy consists of damaged nerves surrounding the skull and the cranium.

These nerves control functions such as hearing, vision, facial movement and other organ's actions. In most cases, Cranial Neuropathy is a secondary condition that results from other medical conditions such as Diabetes.

Cranial Neuropathy may be caused by conditions such as Sarcoidosis, Lyme's Disease and HIV infection. The symptoms of Cranial Neuropathy may clear after some months but may be permanent in some cases.

The symptoms in this condition vary significantly depending on the nerves affected.

In most cases, one of the most common damages occurs in the facial nerve which results in facial pain and eye muscle paralysis. Additionally, this condition has other complications such as twitches, Bell's Palsy, and facial tics.

Treatment of the conditions may range from treating the cause, to use of anti-inflammatory drugs and use of eye ointments among others.

Autonomic Neuropathy

Autonomic Neuropathy is a nerve disorder caused by autoimmune diseases, amyloidosis (abnormal protein buildup), Parkinson's Disease, nerve injury, hereditary disorders and some types of drugs used in the treatment of cancer i.e. chemotherapy.

It affects the parts of the body that are not under your conscious control such as the heart rate, digestion, perspiration and blood pressure.

Although it is not known as a specific disease, it is often referred or associated with damage to autonomic nerves.

The different types of Neuropathy described should be verified with your chosen physician.

For a complete diagnosis, please contact a physician to get started towards maintaining and keeping great health. The overall results are priceless!

Chapter 5: Neuropathy Symptoms

People suffering from Neuropathy report feeling a tingling or burning sensation at the onset of the disease.

This sensation is similar to the sensation felt when one wears a thin stocking or glove.

Neuropathy symptoms depend on the type of Neuropathy and type of nerves affected. The nerves that reach the toes are affected first because the condition affects the longest nerves first.

Sensory nerve damage has the following symptoms:

- Numbness and tingling sensation in the feet or hands
- Burning pains
- Sharp pains
- Acute sensitivity to touch
- Noticeable changes on the skin, nail, or hair
- Poor coordination

Neuropathy Symptoms

Symptoms of Neuropathy of the motor nerves may include

- Muscle weakness
- Complete paralysis

Typical symptoms of Autonomic Nerve Neuropathy are:

- Heat intolerance
- Digestive problems
- Dizziness caused by changes in blood pressure

Diabetic patients suffering from Diabetic Neuropathy are often asymptomatic. However, healthcare professionals can identify slight tell-tale signs of the condition in the form of reduced ankle reflexes and painless foot injuries.

Patients report pain in the toes, feet, or legs that can be either "stabbing" or "burning".

This pain is severe and troublesome at night leading to loss of sleep or troubled sleep.

Smaller nerves produce burning like pain while larger ones produce electric tingling sensation.

Symptoms of Diabetic Neuropathy are distinguishable through the types of nerves involved.

Diabetic Neuropathy caused by autonomic nerves produce the following symptoms:

- Abnormal heart effects such as heart beating too fast or Tachycardia
- Urinary problems
- Sexual problems

- Low blood pressure when standing up

Physicians look out for following Diabetic Neuropathy symptoms:

- Reduced ankle reflexes
- Infections
- Gangrene
- Painless injuries

Persons exhibiting these symptoms should immediately consult a doctor for medical check-up.

Because Diabetic Neuropathy is common with diabetic patients, regular examination of the disease is advisable.

Chapter 6: Managing and Treating Neuropathy Symptoms

For diabetics and those suffering from the debilitating effects of other diseases and health conditions, (e.g., kidney and liver disease, cancer, Lyme's Disease, etc.), Neuropathy is one of the most vexing and difficult complications to treat and manage.

Defined as nerve damage in the peripheral nervous system, symptoms normally begin with a tingling or burning sensation in the feet and hands, which often spreads to the legs and arms.

More severe symptoms include pain, muscle weakness or paralysis, blood pressure issues, and heart, digestive or sexual problems.

While there is no universal cure for Neuropathy, there are a variety of non-invasive, effective treatments to help manage pain and improve function:

Transcutaneous Electrical Nerve Stimulation (TENS)

In this form of treatment, electrodes are attached to the skin using an adhesive and a gentle current is delivered to the affected areas at varying frequencies.

TENS is normally performed daily for a half hour over a period of 30 days, with some patients reporting pain relief and increased feeling and sensation from the therapy.

Massage Therapy

For many with Diabetes or chemotherapy-induced Neuropathy massage therapy has been shown to be one of the most effective ways to manage and reduce pain, and the protocol used by massage therapists is an excellent way to monitor symptoms.

The protocol begins with examining the feet, looking for sores, redness, cracks in the skin, toenail fungus (common on cancer patients) and dark spots (gas gangrene first appears in this form).

Therapists then begin with light pressure, charting the patient's pain response, working from the feet or hands up to the ankle, legs, wrists and arms.

Performed once a week, massage therapy can also help restore range of motion, improve circulation and stimulate nerves, and the self-massage techniques that many therapists teach patients can lead to improvement as well.

Physical Therapy

PT doesn't cure Neuropathy, although there are instances in which physical therapists have been able to eliminate entrapment Neuropathy by freeing the trapped nerve.

It can help with muscle weakness or atrophy, though, and it can also improve strength, balance, coordination and flexibility.

Topical Creams

The advantage of these kinds of creams is that they can be applied directly to the pain site, where they act as local anesthetics, numbing the site to provide relief.

Many of these products contain capsaicin, a painkiller derived from chili peppers, while others use botanical oils.

There is also a medical grade topical cream available from my office which relies on a menthol base and is very effective.

Neuropathy Support Supplements

This is a broad category that includes both supplements as well as holistic and dietary approaches to managing Neuropathy.

The most common is a formula that combines alpha lipoic acid, benfotiamine and methylcobalamine in a single, natural herbal product.

Other promising possibilities include B12 shots (which can actually cure Neuropathy if it is caused by a severe B12 deficiency), acetyl-L-carnitine, and gamma linolenic acid.

Herbal approaches include curcumin, geranium oil, evening primrose oil, and fish oil supplements with omega-3 fatty acids.

In a later chapter I outline more of the helpful vitamins and herbs in more detail.

The nutritional approach seems most effective when combined with other treatments.

Mechanical and Vertical Sound Vibration

This is yet another broad category that includes several innovative approaches.

There is some evidence that applying low-level mechanical or electrical noise to the skin of healthy subjects and older adults can significantly enhance tactile sensitivity.

Stimulation is applied to the foot, being careful to establish and observe a sensitivity threshold.

The mechanisms behind improvement aren't fully understood, but this kind of noise may add mechanical energy that enhances vibration transmission through the dermal tissue.

It may also change the so-called "pain gate" in the spinal cord to help with nerve function and restore tactile sensitivity.

Sound vibration is an analogous technique that has also been effective treating auditory

Neuropathy, which occurs when sound enters the inner ear but signals from the inner ear to the brain are impaired due to damage to inner hair cells.

The treatment involves standing on a vibrating platform, which activates body's stretch reflex for spontaneous muscle contraction, with the rest allowing the body to recover enough to sometimes restore function.

I use both of these techniques in my office to good effect.

Infrared Light Therapy

Light therapy using infrared LEDs has been effective as a general treatment across the spectrum of different types of Neuropathy and symptoms.

An LED light "boot" or blanket is used on the effected areas and stimulates the blood circulation. This releases nitric oxide which in turn aids in the healing of the nerves.

Laser Therapy

One of the most recent breakthroughs in the treatment of Neuropathy is the use of a specially designed warm laser.

I have found this to be the most effective of the various treatments.

These warm laser mcdical devices are FDA approved and are used on the surface of the skin. The special laser light stimulates the deep tissue and provides both relief from pain and stimulates healing.

Chapter 7: Natural Options for Handling the Symptoms of Neuropathy

According to a report released by the Neuropathy Association an estimated 20 million individuals suffer from mild to severe forms of Neuropathy.

This painful and debilitating condition can significantly decrease a patient's quality of life and can result in serious complications including foot ulcers, cardiac arrhythmias, and death.

There are numerous medications that are used to control the symptoms of Neuropathy, but there are also natural supplements that have been proven to reduce the symptoms without the side effects associated with many medications.

Benfotiamine

Benfotiamine is a man-made form of vitamin B1(also known as thiamine), a vitamin that is essential for nerves to function properly.

Taking a vitamin B1 supplement ensures that the body has adequate levels of B1 in it which can result in a decrease in the symptoms of Neuropathy.

It has been shown to be particularly effective in decreasing pain associated with Diabetic Neuropathy and it also reduces microvascular damage that results from frequent high blood sugar levels.

Vitamin B2

Vitamin B2 (also known as riboflavin) is an antioxidant that works to make certain the nervous system is properly functioning and fights off free radicals in the body that cause pain.

Physicians have found that having a deficient amount of vitamin B2 can lead to or worsen the symptoms of Peripheral Neuropathy.

Vitamin B6

Vitamin B6 (commonly called pyridoxone) is an essential vitamin that is required in sufficient levels for fat, carbohydrate, and protein metabolism.

Deficient levels in the body can result in fatigue, moodiness, irritability, and Neuropathy.

Researchers have found that almost all diabetics suffering from Neuropathy have a vitamin B6 deficiency resulting in worsening symptoms.

As a result supplementation provides the amount the body requires and symptoms of Neuropathy decrease.

Vitamin B12

Vitamin B12 (also referred to as methylcobalamine) is necessary to protect the body against neurological diseases.

High levels of methylcobalamine have been proven to regenerate neurons and the myelin sheath that provides protection for the nerve axons and peripheral nerves.

Patients that have received injections of vitamin B12 in the form of methylcobalamine have reported decreased Neuropathy symptoms as well as improved balance and less weakness.

Vitamin D

Vitamin D promotes nerve and neuron growth. Deficient levels of Vitamin D have been determined to impair pain receptor function, increase the potential for nerve damage, and to be a risk factor for Diabetic Neuropathy.

Recent research has found that Vitamin D supplementation can slow down progression of the condition and significantly decreases the amount of neuropathic pain felt.

Vitamin D is usually accompanied by Vitamin A.

R-Alpha Lipoic Acid

R-Alpha Lipoic Acid is an antioxidant

produced by the body and found in all cells.

Studies have shown that its effectiveness at killing free radicals proves beneficial to patients suffering from Peripheral Neuropathy.

Patients who have received this in IV form report decreased burning, tingling, itching, and numbness associated with nerve damage.

It has also decreased symptoms associated with autonomic Neuropathy when taken orally.

The gold standard for alpha lipoic acid treatment is a time released formula, which will provide a constant supply of alpha lipoic acid for the nerves. Most ALA supplements DO NOT contain time released ALA because of the increased cost.

Natural Herbs

There are also numerous herbs available that have proven to be beneficial in the reduction of Neuropathy symptoms.

Feverfew Extract has been found to help control the symptoms of Neuropathy, specifically nerve pain.

Oat Straw Extract acts to decrease general pain, nerve pain, and helps sooth the itchy skin that some patients develop with Neuropathy.

Skullcap Extract works to cause a tranquilizing effect on the nervous system. It has a tremendous impact on decreasing Neuropathy symptoms including pain and tingling.

Finally, Flower Passion is an herb that has been found to eliminate symptoms especially nerve pain. Many patients take more than one supplement for maximum relief.

Before beginning any supplements it is essential to speak with your physician to find out if there may be any possible interactions with your current medicine regimen and to determine what dosages are appropriate for you.

Be aware that most patients report it takes approximately three weeks to begin seeing the benefits associated with taking these supplements.

Chapter 8: Neuropathy Avoidance and Reversing Neuropathy

Neuropathy is a complication which is found in a number of different underlying conditions.

It is damage to the nerves which are outside the central nervous system.

As such it is usually referred to as Peripheral Neuropathy since the nerves it affects are found in the peripheral nervous system.

It is also sometimes referred to as Polyneuropathy because it typically affects multiple nerves simultaneously.

When no underlying cause has been diagnosed, it is referred to as Idiopathic Neuropathy.

As covered earlier, there are a number of factors which lead to Neuropathy including physical trauma, repetitive injury, metabolic problems, and exposure to infections and toxins.

Others are medical conditions such as Diabetes, HIV/AIDS, kidney disease, lymphoma, multiple myeloma, diphtheria and Guillain-Barré syndrome.

Neuropathy affects sensory nerves, motor nerves and involuntary nerves.

Neuropathy Avoidance

Avoiding Neuropathy entails taking measures which limit the conditions which lead to its occurrence. Some of the measures are the following:

Taking care when participating in sports or performing any physical activity.

Any direct injury to a nerve can lead to the emergence of Neuropathy.

Therefore special care should be taken in terms of using protective gear to avoid or mitigate injury.

Treating predisposing medical conditions.

Treating diseases such as Diabetes, kidney disease and the other conditions mentioned earlier.

Patients with these conditions need vigilant treatment and monitoring in order to prevent those conditions from degeneration into Neuropathy.

Taking precaution against getting exposed to toxins or viral infection:

Precautions against toxins include poisons and dysfunctional medicines. The precaution can take the form of avoiding exposure and prompt management in case exposure takes place. Avoid placing repeated pressure on a nerve.

Take daily vitamins to help strengthen the immune system:

Vitamin B-12 in particular is critical in the prevention of Neuropathy. This can be done through eating foods which are rich in Vitamin B-12 or taking Vitamin B-12 supplements.

Reversing Neuropathy

"Reversing" Neuropathy entails taking actions which can reverse the negative effects of Neuropathy. Medically this involves taking steps to eradicate symptoms only.

Yes, that's correct, in medical circles it is typically considered reversed when the symptoms abate. To that end you can expect to be treated with drugs.

Prosthetic Pain: Prosthetic pain can be mitigated using drugs which can mitigate the pain. Such drugs typically include pain killers or pain relief therapies.

The drugs must be prescribed by a doctor for a specific patient; but the common drugs are brand names such as Oxecta, Oxycotin and Cozip. Skin patches containing anesthetics can also be used to relieve the pain.

I am not in favor of drug treatments to handle symptoms. In my office we go for a true reversal, which would be the re-growth of the damaged nerves themselves where possible.

Non Drug Measures: Non-drug measures include wearing garments which can cause minimal irritation, covering sensitive areas with wound dressing and using cold packs.

Such measures are useful for minimizing the discomfort that is results from the condition.

Various Therapies: Other complementary therapies such as stress-relief, meditation, massage, vitamin therapy and relaxation techniques can be used alongside regular treatment.

Such measures will boost a patient's ability to cope with the condition.

Specified Treatment: There are also treatments which are targeted towards strains of Neuropathy which are caused by specific conditions such as Diabetes.

This involves treating the specific ailments such as urinary symptoms, digestive problems, sexual dysfunctions and orthostatic hypotension.

Overall, given the fact that Neuropathy is caused by multiple factors, mitigating and treating it requires multi-faceted approach.

The approaches that are listed are useful for both avoiding and reversing Neuropathy. With the help of a licensed physician that specializes in this area, help is available.

Chapter 9: Neuropathy and Lifestyle

Changes to Make to Reduce or Eliminate Neuropathy Pain and Symptoms

Living with pain everyday is not only uncomfortable, but depressing as well. One common cause for ongoing pain is the condition known as Neuropathy. There are various diseases, which cause painful nerve damage in the human body.

In fact, the medical industry has identified 100 known types of nerve pain. In America today, about 3% of the population suffers from some form of nerve pain and its symptoms. Symptoms include numbness or tingling in the extremities, the degree of which can range from moderate to severe.

The sufferer may experience painful pins and needles sensations in the feet or hands and fingers.

Feelings of intense heat or cold due to decreased circulation in the limbs are other symptoms. Ongoing nerve pain is the basis for diagnosing patients with Neuropathy.

The pain and symptoms of Neuropathy can affect one's ability to go about functioning normally in their everyday life.

However, making a few simple lifestyle changes can limit the risk of one's health from spiraling down, due to the pain of living with damaged nerves that can lead to inactivity.

The less active the person is, the more chances chronic pain has to restrict mobility.

The last thing the patient wants is to become bed ridden, so the faster one can make lifestyle changes to reduce or eliminate Neuropathy pain and symptoms, the better chances they have for maintaining a happy and productive life.

Change Your Diet

People living with Neuropathy and its symptoms should begin by changing their diet.

One of the most important diet changes to make is to include more fruits and vegetables. In fact, one should switch over to diet heavy in vegetables.

Eat lots of green leafy vegetables. Be sure to add more of the darker fruits such as blueberries and pomegranates, purple grapes and black plumbs to the diet.

This ensures the body gets enough of the vitamins, minerals and antioxidants it needs to support health and energy levels.

Stop Smoking

Stop the Consumption of Alcohol

Add an Exercise Routine

Exercising is very important. It helps keep the body limber and the muscles strong. Before beginning, take the time to learn how to exercise properly to avoid injury and do not forget to do a warm up before exercising and a cool down afterward.

Get at least two 15 minutes sessions of moderate exercise in each day. Low impact exercises are best, such as walking and swimming.

Wear Loose Clothing and Shoes

Tight socks and shoes can cause poor circulation in the feet and legs. Wear loose-fitting clothes to help reduce pain and symptoms.

Wear the proper footwear that your doctor recommends for people who have Neuropathy pain in the feet.

Eating right, exercising the right way, and wearing the right type of clothing, are important lifestyle changes to make to reduce or eliminate Neuropathy pain and symptoms.

Testimonials

When I first came to the clinic, I could barely walk. Now I can do almost anything: exercising, and dancing... I really recommend Dr. Hashimoto, he is a wonderful doctor.

-Vicki

When I came here, my hands were numb and I had a headache every day. Since that time, my hands are no longer numb and my headaches are gone!

-Marla D.

I am very happy that I am able to walk, because I was not able to walk when I first came in to see Dr. Hashimoto. Now, believe it or not, I am walking without a cane!

-Maria H.

I have been coming to Dr. Hashimoto for almost 2 months because of pain and trouble sleeping. Thanks to Dr. Naota I am no longer in pain, I sleep better, and I can dance now!

-Lernal

Since I have been coming to see Dr. Hashimoto, the pain and numbness in my toes and feet have much improved.

-Jennifer

When I first came to Dr. Hashimoto, I could hardly walk with a cane. Now, I'm ready to go tap dancing and mountain climbing! I really appreciate it!

-Bob

I just finished my first treatment, and I am able to walk. When I first came in here today, I was limping. Now, I have lost my limp.

-Betty

I can walk much better and I feel much better. He has taken very good care of me. Thank you.

-Barbara T.

INDEX